Tayssir Ben Achour

Special features of male systemic lupus erythematosus

Tayssir Ben Achour

Special features of male systemic lupus erythematosus

ScienciaScripts

Imprint

Cover image: www.ingimage.com

This book is a translation from the original published under ISBN 978-620-6-70784-4.

Publisher:
Sciencia Scripts
is a trademark of
Dodo Books Indian Ocean Ltd. and OmniScriptum S.R.L publishing group

120 High Road, East Finchley, London, N2 9ED, United Kingdom
Str. Armeneasca 28/1, office 1, Chisinau MD-2012, Republic of Moldova, Europe
Managing Directors: Ieva Konstantinova, Victoria Ursu
info@omniscriptum.com

Printed at: see last page
ISBN: 978-620-8-62451-4

SPECIFIC FEATURES OF MALE SYSTEMIC LUPUS ERYTHEMATOSUS

PREPARED BY DR TAYSSIR BEN ACHOUR

19-12-2024

CONTENTS

INTRODUCTION

Systemic lupus erythematosus (SLE) is a non-organ-specific autoimmune disease of polymorphous clinical expression. It is characterised by the production of multiple autoantibodies, the most characteristic of which are directed against certain components of the nucleus, such as native deoxyribonucleic acid (DNA) and nucleosomes. These autoantibodies have been shown to play a role in the pathogenesis of the disease, either by binding directly to their target and activating complement, leading to tissue lysis, or via the deposition of circulating immune complexes or complexes formed in situ **[1].** Its aetiopathogenesis is still debated. However, many genetic, endocrine, immunological and environmental factors contribute to the onset and maintenance of this disease **[2].**

SLE tends to affect young women of childbearing age, with a sex ratio of approximately 9 women to 1 man according to several series **[2,3].** Male lupus is rarer but considered more serious and more prone to complications **[4].** In Tunisia, studies of male SLE are few and have involved small numbers of patients **[5].**

The aim of our work is to describe the epidemiological, clinical and paraclinical characteristics of male lupus, as well as the treatment and progression of the disease.

MATERIALS AND METHODS

I. Type of study :

This was a retrospective, descriptive, single-centre study conducted in the internal medicine department of the Hôpital Militaire Principal d'Instruction de Tunis over an 18-year period from 1st January 2000 to 30 June 2018. We collected 21 records of male lupus patients hospitalized during this period.

II. Population studied

We included 21 lupus patients with a diagnosis of SLE according to the classification criteria of the American College of Rheumatology (ACR) revised in 1997 (appendix 1).

1. Inclusion :

✓ Male gender

✓ Age greater than or equal to 16

2. Non-inclusion criteria :

✓ Outpatients with lupus

✓ Female gender

1. Exclusion criteria :

✓ Files that cannot be used

✓ Patients lost to follow-up

III. Ethical considerations

Our study was accepted by the ethics committee of the Faculty of Medicine in Sousse.

IV. Data collection :

1. **Epidemiological, clinical, paraclinical, therapeutic and developmental data:**

The epidemiological, clinical, biological, immunological, radiological, therapeutic and evolutionary characteristics of each lupus patient were collected on a pre-established information sheet.

1.1.Epidemiological data :

✓ The following were identified:

Anamnestic data: age, personal history, family history of autoimmune diseases, mode of onset of the disease, age at onset of the disease, etc.

1.2.Clinical data :

✓ General signs (fever, asthenia, weight loss)

✓ Mucocutaneous manifestations (photosensitivity, malar rash, mouth ulcers, lupus discordata, alopecia, purpura, Raynaud's phenomenon, livedo, etc.).

✓ Rheumatological manifestations (arthralgia, arthritis, myalgia, myositis)

✓ Cardiac manifestations (pericarditis, endocarditis, myocarditis),

✓ Pleuropulmonary manifestations (parenchymal involvement, pleurisy, PAH)

✓ Central and peripheral neurological manifestations

✓ Renal manifestations (proteinuria, haematuria, nephrotic syndrome, oedema, renal failure, recourse to haemodialysis) with data from the renal biopsy.

✓ Digestive disorders (digestive haemorrhage, pancreatitis, etc.)

1.3 Para-clinical data :

1.3.1. Biological tests :

- Blood count (CBC), inflammatory work-up: sedimentation rate (ESR), C Reactive Protein (CRP), fibrinogen, protein electrophoresis (PEE); urinary work-up (creatininaemia, blood urea, 24-hour proteinuria, ECBU).
- Immunological parameters: antinuclear antibodies (ANA), native anti-DNA antibodies, anti-Sm antibodies, anti-SSA antibodies, anti-SSB antibodies, anti-Rnp antibodies, anti-phospholipid antibodies (lupus-type circulating anticoagulant, anti-cardiolipin antibodies, anti-B2 glycoprotein1 antibodies), assay of complement fractions C3 and C4.

1.3.2. Other para-clinical examinations :

Chest x-ray, computer tomography (CT), magnetic resonance imaging (MRI), cardiac ultrasound, electromyogram (EMG), etc.

1.4 Therapeutic management

■ Hygienic and dietary rules.

■ Drugs prescribed: Non-steroidal anti-inflammatory drugs (NSAIDs), synthetic antimalarials (SMAs), corticosteroids (doses, methods, duration), immunosuppressants (cyclophosphamide, azathioprine, mycophenolate mofetil (MMF), methotrexate, biotherapies (anti CD20), etc.).

- **1.5 Future developments**

Complete remissions, stabilisations, complications and deaths have been described. Disease activity was studied by calculating the systemic lupus erythematosus disease activity index (SLEDAI), which was developed in 1992 overall disease activity. It comprises 24 items covering 9 domains, and does not include subjective symptoms. Several modifications of this score have been suggested, but the most widely used is the one proposed for the SELENA trial: SLEDAI-SELENA **(Appendix 2)**.

V. Statistical study :

- Patient data were entered and analysed using Microsoft Excel 2016.
- Statistical analysis was carried out using IBM SPSS Statistics version 21 software. We calculated simple frequencies and relative frequencies (percentages) for the qualitative variables. We calculated means, medians and standard deviations and determined extreme values for quantitative variables.

VI. Bibliographic research :

The bibliography of our work was established by consulting the Medline and Embase databases and the thesis archives of the Tunis Faculty of Medicine. The search engines used were : Pub Med and Sciencedirect

VII. Conflicts interest :

No conflicts of interest need to be declared.

RESULTS

1. Characteristics of the study population :

1.1 Epidemiological characteristics :

1.1.1 Genre :

Our study involved 21 men with SLE.

1.1.2. Age:

The age at onset of lupus disease in the male subjects was 35.2 years, with a standard deviation of 14.1 years and age extremes ranging from 11 to 84 years. The mean age at the time of the study was 37.8 years.

1.1.3. Family history of SLE :

One patient had a family history of SLE.

1.2.Clinical characteristics

1.2.1The inaugural events of the LES :

In our series, rheumatological manifestations were indicative of SLE in 10 patients (47.6% of cases). Figure 1 shows the frequency of the different inaugural manifestations of SLE in the patients in our series.

1.2.2. General signs

General signs were observed in 10 patients (47.6% of cases). A fever of 38-38.5 with no infectious cause was present in 8 patients (38.1%). Weight loss was observed in two patients (9.5%) and asthenia in one

(4.8%).

1.2.3. Mucocutaneous manifestations

Mucocutaneous involvement was observed in 17 patients (81%). Photosensitivity and malar rash were found respectively in 11 and 10 patients in our series (52.4% and 47.6%). Raynaud's syndrome was present in 4 patients (19%). Vascular purpura was noted in 3 patients (14.3%) and one patient had lupus discordans (4.8%). The frequency of the various cutaneous and mucosal manifestations is shown in Figure 2.

1.2.4. Manifestations of the musculoskeletal system :

Inflammatory-type arthralgias were noted in all patients. Asymmetric polyarthralgia affecting large and small joints was present in all cases. Non-destructive, non-deforming arthritis was observed in 6 patients (28.6% of cases). Myalgias were present in 4 patients (19%). Myositis was present in 2 patients (9.5%). Table I summarises the rheumatological manifestations of our patients.

Table I: Rheumatological symptoms in our patients

Arthralgia	21 (100%)
Arthritis	6 (28,6%)
Myalgias	4 (19%)
Myositis	2 (9,5%)

1.2.5. Kidney disorders

Fifteen patients had renal involvement (71.4% of cases). Clinically, three patients (14.3%) presented with white, soft, renal-like oedema.4 (19%) had hypertension.13 (61.9%) patients had positive proteinuria, associated with nephrotic syndrome in 4 (19%).Seven (33.3%) patients had microscopic haematuria. Renal failure was observed in nine patients (42.9% of cases), with haemodialysis in five cases (23.8% of cases). Table II shows the different clinico-biological presentations of renal involvement in our series.

Table II: Different clinico-biological presentations kidney damage

HTA	4 (19%)
Haematuria	7 (33,3%)
Proteinuria	13 (61,9%)
Edema	3 (14,3%)
Nephrotic syndrome	4 (19%)
Renal insufficiency	9 (42,9%)
Haemodialysis	5 (23,8%)

A renal biopsy was performed in 10 cases, showing 5 cases of class IV lupus nephropathy, 3 class III cases, 1 class V case and one class I case.

1.2.6 Cardiac manifestations

In our series, 10 patients (47.6%) had cardiac involvement. Cardiac ultrasonography was performed in all patients, and pericarditis was observed in 42.9% of cases. Figure 2 shows an aortic leak on colour

Doppler in one patient in our series.

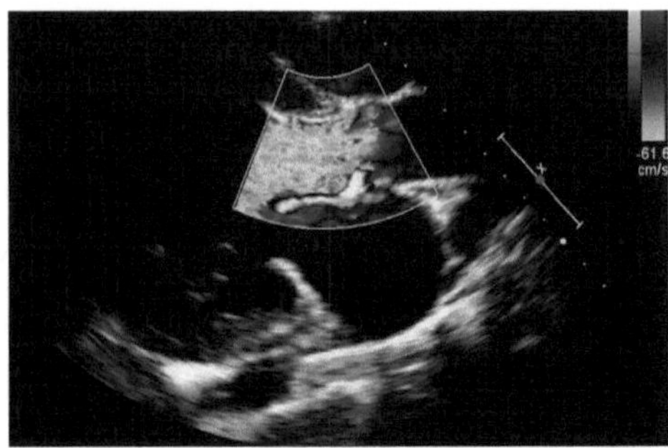

The different cardiac manifestations of these patients are presented in Table III.

Table III: Cardiac manifestations in men with lupus

Cardiac	10 (47,6%)
Chest pain	7 (33,3%)
Palpitations	1 (4,8%)
Dyspnoea	8 (38 1%)
Pericarditis	9 (42 9%)
Myocarditis	1 (4 8%)
Endocarditis	0
Valvulopathy	6 (28 6%)

1.2.7 Pleuropulmonary manifestations

Twelve patients (57.1%) had pulmonary involvement. Pleural effusion was observed in 6 patients (28.6%), pulmonary arterial hypertension in 3 patients (14.3%), and diffuse interstitial lung disease in 3 cases. The combination of pericarditis and pleural effusion was observed in 5 cases (23.8%).

Table IV summarises the pleural and pulmonary disorders in our patients.

Table IV: Pleuropulmonary disorders in our patients

PAH	3 (14,3%)
Pleuresis	6 (28,6%)
Interstitial lung disease	3 (14,3%)

1.2.8Neuropsychiatric manifestations

Neuropsychiatric manifestations of central origin were found in 4 patients (19% of cases). Cognitive disorders such as confusion were observed in 3 patients (14.3%). Figure 3 shows parenchymal neurological involvement on brain MRI in a 17-year-old patient who presented with a generalised tonic-clonic seizure.

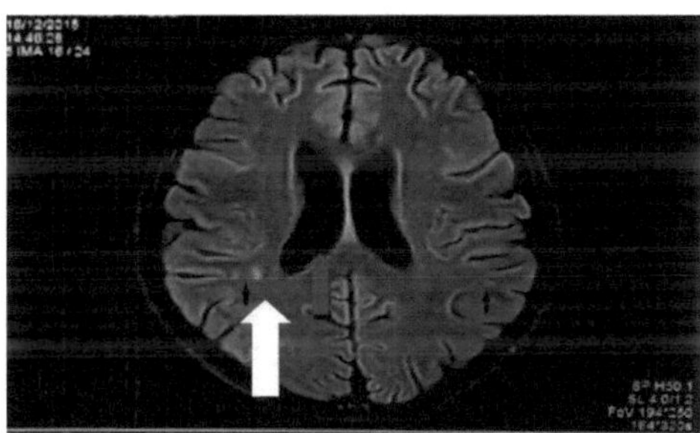

Figure 3: Axial section of a brain MRI scan showing subcortical demyelinating lesions in T2 Flair hypersignal.

Peripheral neuropathy was observed in four cases (19%).

1.2.9 Haematological manifestations

Haematological manifestations were observed in 13 patients in our series (61.9% of cases). Two patients had developed macrophagic activation syndrome during the course of the disease. Three patients had an Evans syndrome combining autoimmune haemolytic anaemia and peripheral thrombocytopenia.

Table V summarises the various haematological disorders found in our series.

Table V: Haematological disorders found in our series

Anemia	13 (61,9%)
Autoimmune haemolytic anaemia	4 (19%)
Thrombocytopenia	8 (38,1%)
Lymphopenia	4 (19%)
Leukopenia	9 (42,85%)

1.2.10Digestive disorders

Five patients in our series (23.8% of cases) had digestive symptoms. Abdominal pain was present in 5 patients (23.8%), and one patient (4.8%) presented with watery diarrhoea; there were no cases of digestive haemorrhage or pancreatitis.

Paraclinical characteristics :

1.3.1. Biological abnormalities :

At the time of the study, 16 patients (76%) had a biological inflammatory syndrome. CRP was > 50 mg/l in six cases (28.5%). The sedimentation rate at the first hour was elevated in 17 patients (80% of cases).

1.3.2. Immunological abnormalities :

All patients in our series were tested for and assayed for NAA. They were positive in 19 patients, i.e. 90.5% of cases. Table VI describes the immunological abnormalities of men with lupus.

Table VI: Distribution of patients according to immunological abnormalities.

AA+	19 (90,5%)
anti DNA +	15 (71,4%)
antiS+	8 (38,1%)
antiSS+	7 (33,3%)
antiSSB+	1 (4,8%)
C3 decreases	9 (45%)
C4 decreases	9 (45%)
anti cardiolipins	1 (4,8%)
anti B2Gp1	0

1.4. Therapeutic management :

11.4.1 Synthetic antimalarials (SMAs) :

PSAs were prescribed for all patients.

1.4.2 Corticosteroids :

Systemic corticosteroid therapy was prescribed in 18 patients (85.7%). It was initiated by methylprednisolone boli in 10 patients (47.6%).

1.4.3 Immunosuppressants :

Immunosuppressive drugs were prescribed in 16 lupus patients (76.1%). These patients had presented with severe visceral damage, such as active proliferative lupus nephropathy, neurolupus or cardiac damage, or had developed cortico-resistance or cortico-dependence.

Table VII: Different treatments administered to our patients

Corticoids	18 (85,7%)
Bolus 1g/d x 3d	10 (47,6%)
10-20 mg/d	0
0.5 mg/kg/day	2 (9,5%)
1 mg/kg/day	15 (71,4%)
Synthetic antimalarials	21 (100%)
Cyclophosphamide	7 (33,3%)
Azathioprine	4 (19%)
Mycophenolate Mofetil	4 (19%)
Anti cd 20	1(4,8%)

1.5. Evolution :

1.5.1 Disease activity (SLEDAI) at the time of study :

Fifteen male patients (71.4%) had a SLEDAI score greater than or equal to 11, i.e. high to very high disease activity. Table VIII summarises the level of disease activity in our patients.

Table VIII: Level disease activity in our patients

SLEDAI score	Level of activity	Gender Male
Between 1 and 5	Light activity	2 (9,5%)
Between 6 and 10	Average activity	4 (19%)
Between 11 and 19	High activity	11 (52,4%)
• 20	Very high activity	4 (19%)

1.5.2 Infectious complications :

Eleven patients (52.4%) had infectious complications. Four patients (5.25%) had developed a viral infection. Three were infected with varicella zoster virus (VZV). One patient had been infected with cytomegalovirus (CMV). In all cases, it was a viral reactivation. Three patients had developed a pulmonary infection, one of which was caused by klebsiella pneumoniae . One patient had orchiepididymitis. One patient had salmonella septicaemia and another alkaligenes Xyloxidans septicaemia. Two patients had presented with tuberculosis, one multifocal and the other pulmonary. Two patients had oropharyngeal candidiasis and one patient had pulmonary aspergillosis. All patients had a favourable outcome, except for one man developed hypoxaemic infectious pneumonitis.

1.5.3 Drug complications :

The drug complications experienced by our patients are summarised in Table IX.

Table IX: Drug complications in our patients

Complications	Patients
Osteopenia	1 (4,8%)
Aseptic osteonecrosis	2 (9,5%)
Oculotoxicity to PSA	1 (4,8%)

DISCUSSION

I Epidemiological data :

I.1. the genre :

Systemic lupus erythematosus is mainly a disease of adult women, rarely affecting men. The female/male sex ratio varies in the literature from 5.8:1 **[1]** to 19.2:1 **[3]**. Due to the nature of Particular to the population studied in our series (military population), the male gender was quite significant.

I.2. Age:

The mean age of patients in our study was 35.2 years, compared with 48.9 years in the Rees study **[1].**

I.2 Family history of lupus :

Familial SLE is rare. Its frequency varies from 4 to 12% according to studies **[4]**. In our series, only one patient a family history of lupus. In 2003, a multicentre study by the Tunisian Society of Internal Medicine found a family history of SLE in 2% of patients **[5]**.

I. Clinical manifestations :

The clinical expression of SLE is polymorphous, affecting several organs to varying degrees

I.1. Clinical manifestations of SLE:

In our series, the manifestations of SLE were varied. Rheumatological manifestations, mainly arthralgias, the most frequent mode of onset.

They were present in 47.6% of patients at the start of the disease. These were followed by mucocutaneous and renal manifestations, which occurred in 19% of patients. General signs were present at the onset of SLE in 9.5% of cases. These results are not consistent with those of a 2016 study of 61 lupus patients **[6]**. In this study, general signs were the most frequent mode of onset: Asthenia and fever were found at the onset of SLE in 91.8% and 88.5% of patients respectively. Arthralgias were present in 90.2% of patients.

II.2 General signs :

General signs are fairly common in SLE. They usually reflect the progressive nature of the disease. Fever and asthenia are the most common signs. As fever is the most frequent sign, it prompts a search for infectious complications, which are very common in this condition. In the literature, its frequency varies between 36% and 86% **[7].** In our series, it was found in 38.1% of patients. In our series, asthenia was noted in 4.8% of patients. It must be distinguished from asthenia due to other factors or intercurrent pathologies. In a series published by Gaüzère et al in 2018, asthenia was found in 72% of patients **[8]**. Weight loss was reported in 9.5% of patients in our series. In the same series by Gaüzère, weight loss was noted in 30% of patients **[8]**. Weight gain may be observed during the course of the disease. This is essentially due to the use of corticosteroids **[9].**

II. 3. Mucocutaneous manifestations :

Mucocutaneous involvement in male lupus is common. They are found in 80% of patients and can occur at any stage of the disease. In 25% of these patients, it is the first sign of SLE **[10]**. In our series, mucocutaneous manifestations were noted in 81% of patients. Our result are in line with those reported in the literature. In a multicentre Tunisian series conducted by S. Othmani et al, male subjects developed less alopecia **[11]**. In the cohort of Tan et al, which included 1979 patients, 157 of whom were male, men developed significantly fewer cutaneous manifestations (malar rash, photosensitivity, Raynaud's phenomenon, oral ulceration, alopecia) **[12]**.

II.4.Rheumatological symptoms :

Rheumatological manifestations in male SLE are frequent. They are inaugural in more than half of cases and are found in 95% of patients during the course of the disease **[13]**. most common symptoms are inflammatory joint pain affecting both large and small joints, sparing the spine. In our series, arthralgia was present in 100% of patients, and was associated with arthritis in 28.6% of patients. It is more frequent according to the literature **[12, 14, 15]** Muscle damage may be associated with joint damage in SLE, leading to increased functional discomfort **[16]**. In the majority of cases, this muscular damage is manifested by simple myalgias or associated with myositis.

In our study, muscle involvement was less frequent than in the literature. Myalgias occurred in around 19% of patients, and myositis was found in 9.5%. A review of the literature had shown that Muscle weakness and myalgia are present in 70% of lupus patients. Myositis is described in 7 to 15% of cases **[13]**.

II.5. Kidney damage :

Lupus nephropathy in humans is one of the most frequent and serious manifestations of SLE. It determines the therapeutic choices made and the vital prognosis of patients. The clinical picture is pleomorphic, ranging from asymptomatic proteinuria to rapidly progressive glomerulonephritis. progressive. In our series, lupus nephropathy was found 71.of patients. Progression to end-stage renal failure with recourse to haemodialysis was noted in 23.8% of patients. In the cohort of Tan**[12]** et al, which included 1979 patients, 157 of whom were male, men developed significantly more renal manifestations (proteinuria, haematuria, nephrotic syndrome, renal failure). Similarly, in a series by Borba et al**[14]**, renal impairment was more frequent in men.

II.6. Cardiovascular symptoms :

Cardiac involvement in SLE can involve all three tunics, the heart valves and the coronary arteries. Pericarditis remains the It may be latent and may be associated with pleurisy. In a series by Tan al, pericarditis was present in 25% of patients **[12]**; in our study, pericarditis was more frequent, occurring in 42.9% of patients. The incidence of myocarditis was around 4.8%. There were no cases of Libman Sacks endocarditis in our series.

II.7. Pleuropulmonary manifestations :

Pleuropulmonary involvement in SLE is less common other systemic manifestations. Its prevalence is estimated at 30% in lupus patients **[19-20], and** is dominated by pleurisy, but it may also manifest as diffuse interstitial lung disease or alveolar haemorrhage. In our series, pulmonary manifestations were noted in 57.1% of patients. Pleural involvement and diffuse interstitial lung disease were found in 28.6 and 14.3% of patients respectively. These results are in line with those reported in the literature **[14,17].** Pulmonary arterial hypertension is a rare complication of SLE, its prevalence varying from 0.5 to 17.5% of cases **[17].** In our series, PAH was found in 14.3% of patients.

II.8. Neuropsychiatric manifestations :

Neuropsychiatric manifestations in SLE are diverse and vary in frequency from 18% to 37% depending on the series **[5,18]**. Involvement of the central nervous system is more frequent than that of the peripheral nervous system. In our series, cognitive disorders were present in 14.3% of cases, convulsions in 4.3% and peripheral neuropathy in 19%.

II.9. Digestive disorders :

The prevalence of digestive damage in male SLE is between 25 and 40%, and is most often inherent to the therapeutic methods or the infections intercurrent infections **[21]**.The symptoms is dominated by the pain nausea, vomiting, diarrhoea and digestive haemorrhage. bleeding. In our series, digestive manifestations were present in 23.of patients. This figure is in line with the literature **[22]**.

II.10. Haematological manifestations :

Haematological manifestations are extremely frequent in SLE. All three blood lines may be affected, but anaemia is the most common, with prevalence varying between 52% and 75% depending on the study **[5, 22, 23]**. 3 to 26% of cases of this anaemia may be haemolytic **[5, 8, 14, 22, 24]**. The mechanism of anaemia must be determined in order institute appropriate treatment. Lymphopenia is present in 26-75% of lupus patients thrombocytopenia is often latent during LES, regardless of gender, and its prevalence varies between 15 and 25% **[2, 6, 14, 22]**.In our series, anaemia was present in 61.9% of patients, and was haemolytic in 19% of cases. Lymphopenia and thrombocytopenia occurred in 19% and 38.1% respectively. In the cohort by Tan et al, men developed haematological disorders (lymphopenia and thrombocytopenia) more frequently than women **[23]**.

The abnormalities immunological abnormalities:

In the series by AI Renau et al, male subjects had a significantly higher frequency of Ig Manti cardiolipins **[15]**. In the cohort by Tan et al, a significantly greater positivity of native anti-Sm and anti-DNA antibodies, as well as a more significant drop in the C3 fraction of complement were noted in male subjects **[12]**. In the results of the Meta-Analysis by Boodhoo et al, the frequency of native anti-DNA antibodies was significantly higher in men, that of AAN antibodies and the fall in the C3 fraction of complement were significantly lower in the same subjects **[17]**.

The table below compares the immunological profile patients in our series with that found in various studies.

	Our series	E.Borba et al [14]	L.Gaüzère et Al [8]	B.Louzir et al [5]
AAN	95,8%	100%	99%	92%
Native DNA antibodies	64,9%	35,1%	70%	74%
Anti Sm	31,9%	21,8%	37%	57%
Ac anti SSA	37,6%	31,6%	47%	52%
SSB antibody	6,5%	7%	24%	34%
C3 and C4 decrease	C3 : 44,3 %C4 : 44,8%	--	53%	C3 : 61% C4 : 75%

IV. Therapeutic management :

Treatment of SLE depends on the organ affected and the severity of the symptoms. It can range from local treatment for cutaneous forms, or a course of NSAIDs for rheumatological conditions, to aggressive immunosuppressive therapy **[22]**.

IV.1. Non-steroidal anti-inflammatory drugs (NSAIDs):

They are used in mild forms of SLE, particularly for minor joint involvement. This explains the low number of patients on NSAIDs in our series (3 patients, i.e. 3.1%), as these were patients hospitalised for more serious symptoms. In the series by L. Gaüzère et al, NSAID treatment was prescribed in 19% of patients **[8]**.

IV.2. Synthetic antimalarials :

The immunomodulatory properties of this therapeutic class mean that it can be used to treat both cutaneous and articular forms of the disease. In our series, all patients (100%) received PSA treatment. This percentage is similar to that in the series by L. Gaüzère et al, which was 98% **[8]**.

IV.3. Corticosteroids :

This is the category most commonly used to treat acute forms of SLE. The dose and route administration vary according to the severity of the disease. the disease and the organs affected **[22]**. In our series, long-term corticosteroid therapy was prescribed in 85.7% of patients.

IV.4.Immunosuppressants :

They are used in severe visceral forms SLE, particularly renal forms, but also in cortico-resistant forms. The table below compares the frequency of use of immunosuppressants in patients with of our series and the series by L.Gaüzère and Al

Immunosuppressants	Our series (%)	L.Gaüzère et al [8] (%)
Cyclophosphamide	21 (100%)	23
Azathioprine	7 (33,3%)	28
Methotrexate	4 (19%)	28
MMF	4 (19%)	24

V. The evolving profile :

V.1. Disease activity: SLEDAI :

The SLEDAI score was used in the patients in our series to assess the level of disease activity. Fifteen male patients (71.4%) had a SLEDAI score greater than or equal to 11, i.e. high to very high disease activity. These results are consistent with those of the series by R. Cervera et al, where the mean SLEDAI score was higher in males and the percentage of patients with a SLEDAI score greater than 10 was also higher in males

V.2. Infectious complications :

Infection is one of the main causes of mortality in SLE. Several factors predispose to infectious complications, such as the lupus disease itself, but also the therapies used **[24]**. In our series, 11 patients (52.4%) developed at least one infectious episode. This result is in line with the frequency of infections in SLE described in the literature: 44.5% in the Tunisian series by M.Jallouli et al **[4]**, and 32.05% in the Moroccan series by K.Echchil ali et al **[24]**. In this study, a lupus patient on immunosuppressants died of rapidly progressive hypoxaemic infectious pneumonitis.

V.3. Non-infectious complications :

These complications are essentially the side-effects of the therapies used. Bone damage and cortico-induced diabetes are the most common complications. The table below compares the frequency of some of these complications in our series and in the series by L.Gaüzère et al **[8]**.

	Our series (%)	L.Gaüzère et Al (%)
Osteoporosis	4,8	5,7
[illegible]	9,5	2,4

V.4. Progression :

The course of the disease in our series was marked by complete remission in 47.6% of patients. The survival rate was 95.2%. In the series by R. Cervera et al, analysis of the percentages of patients who developed relapses showed no significant differences between patients of the two genders **[3]**. Several published studies also report a poorer prognosis for male lupus patients **[15]**. In the series by Tan et al, mortality was significantly higher in male patients **[12]**.

VI. Limits of the study

This was a descriptive study, not a comparison between the two genera.

VII. Benefits of study

The major interest of our study was to deepen our knowledge of lupus in Tunisian men. Given the particularity of the population in our series (military population), we had a good number of male patients.

VIII. Outlook

This study could form part of a national multicentre study aimed at studying the particularities of SLE in men in Tunisia.

	Our series		Borba et al [14]	AI Renau et al [15]	Tan et al [12]
	%	%	%	%	%
Malaria rash	52,4	71	69,4	64,4	39,7
Photosensitivity	47,6	41	75	35,6	40,4
Raynaud's disease	19	26			35,7
Oral ulcers	4,8	12,5	15,3	13,3	34
Alopecia	0	12,5		15,6	28,2
Joint damage	66,7	95	88,9	93,3	87,3
Pericarditis	42,9	37,5	11,1		25
Pleuresis	28,6	20	25		41,7
Haemolytic anaemia	19	12,5	5,6	4,4	12,8
Lymphopenia	19	46	30,6	84,4	49,4
Thrombocytopenia	38,1	12,5	15,3	11,1	28,8
Kidney damage	71,4	66	47,2	31,1	
Renal insufficiency	42,9	12,5		4,4	34,1
CNS damage	19	12,5	8,3	26,7	
Peripheral neuropathy	19	0			

CONCLUSION

Lupus erythematosus (SLE) is an autoimmune disease that affects women particular, but rarely occurs men. A few studies have investigated the specific features of male lupus. There are major clinical differences between male and female lupus. Male SLE is known to be more prone to complications.

In our series of male lupus patients, the most frequent manifestations of SLE were rheumatological, present in 47.6% of patients, followed by mucocutaneous and renal manifestations in 19% of patients.

Clinical analysis of the patients in our series enabled us to determine the disorders most frequently developed during the course of male SLE: rheumatological manifestations mainly arthralgia) were present in all patients, followed mucocutaneous manifestations (mainly malar rash and photosensitivity), which were present in 81% of patients. Renal involvement was present in 71.4% of patients. There was a high prevalence of cardiac and pleural manifestations in men. Fifteen male patients (71.4%) had a SLEDAI score of 11 or above, representing high to very high disease activity. Infectious complications were dominated by pneumopathies and urinary tract infections. Non-infectious complications were essentially undesirable effects of treatment, particularly corticosteroids. A multicentre study involving a larger number of lupus-affected men would be a project for another study to provide a more precise picture of the characteristics of male SLE in Tunisia.

REFERENCES

1. Meyer O. Systemic lupus erythematosus. EMC - Rheumatology-Orthopaedics. Jan 2005; 2(1):1-32.

2. Cervera R, Doria A, Amoura Z, Khamashta M, Schneider M, Guillemin F, et al. Patterns of systemic lupus erythematosus expression in Europe. Autoimmunity Reviews. June 2014;13(6):621-9

3. Vila LM. Early clinical manifestations, disease activity and damage of systemic lupus erythematosus among two distinct US Hispanic subpopulations. Rheumatology. 16 Dec 2003;43(3):358-63.

4. Jallouli M, Frigui M, Marzouk S, Mâaloul I, Kaddour N, Bahloul Z. Infectious complications in systemic lupus erythematosus: a study of 146 patients. La Revue de Médecine Interne. August 2008;29(8):626-31.

5. Louzir B, Othmani S, Ben Abdelhafidh N. Systemic lupus erythematosus in Tunisia. National multicentre study. About 295 observations. La Revue de Médecine Interne. Dec 2003;24(12):768-74.

6. Batool S, Ahmad NM, Saeed MA, Farman S. Pattern of initial clinical manifestations of systemic lupus erythematosus in a tertiary care hospital. Pakistan Journal of Medical Sciences [Internet]. 19 Sep 2016 [cited 3 Mar 2019];32(5).

7. Timlin H, Syed A, Haque U, Adler B, Law G, Machireddy K, et al. Fevers in Adult Lupus Patients. Cureus. 22 Jan 2018.

8. Gaüzère, L., Gerber, A., Renou, F., Ferrandiz, D., Bagny, K.,

Osdoit, S., Yvin, J. and Raffray, L. (2018). Characteristics of systemic lupus erythematosus in La Réunion: a retrospective study in the adult population at the CHU of Saint-Denis. La Revue de Médecine Interne.

9. Fortuna G, Brennan MT. Systemic Lupus Erythematosus. Dental Clinics of North America. oct 2013;57(4):631-55.

10. Doffoel-Hantz V, Savi V. Main dermatological manifestations of systemic lupus erythematosus. Pharmaceutical News. june 2017;56(567):22-5.

11. Othmani S, Louzir B. Systemic lupus in 24 Tunisian men: clinicobiological and evolutionary analysis. La Revue de Médecine Interne. Dec 2002;23(12):983-90.

12. Tan TC, Fang H, Magder LS, Petri MA. Differences between Male and Female Systemic Lupus Erythematosus in a Multiethnic Population. The Journal of Rheumatology. Apr 2012;39(4):759-69.

13. Dernis E, Puéchal X. Articular and muscular manifestations of lupus. Revue du Rhumatisme. Feb 2005;72(2):150-4.

14. Borba E, Araujo D, Bonfá E, Shinjo S. Clinical and immunological features of 888 Brazilian systemic lupus patients from a monocentric cohort: comparison with other populations. Lupus. June 2013;22(7):744-9.

15. Renau A, Isenberg D. Male versus female lupus: a comparison of ethnicity, clinical features, serology and outcome over a 30 years period. Lupus. Sept 2012;21(10):1041-8.

16. Ben Yahia W, Atig A, Bouker A, Zallema D, Zaglaoui H, Nouira R, et al. Muscle involvement during systemic Lupus erythematosus.

La Revue de Médecine Interne. June 2018;39:A235-6.

17. Boodhoo KD, Liu S, Zuo X. Impact of sex disparities on the clinical manifestations in patients with systemic lupus erythematosus: A systematic review and meta-analysis. Medicine. Jul 2016;95(29):e4272.

18. Kado R. Systemic Lupus Erythematosus for Primary Care. Primary Care: Clinics in Office Practice. June 2018;45(2):257-70.

19. Klii R, Chaabene I, Bennasr M, Kechida M, Hammami S, Jguirim M, et al. Pulmonary involvement during systemic lupus erythematosus. Revue des Maladies Respiratoires. Jan 2018;35:A119.

20. Oubelkacem N, Khammar Z, Hamri L, Atik S, Khoussar I, Ouazzani M, et al. Lung involvement during systemic lupus: is it a mortality factor? La Revue de Médecine Interne. June 2016;37:A77.

21. Harouna H, Bouissar W, Echchilali K, Moudatir M, Alaoui F, El Kabli H. Digestive involvement during systemic lupus erythematosus. Revue du Rhumatisme. nov 2016;83:A185.

22. Yeoh S-A, Dias SS, Isenberg DA. Advances in systemic lupus erythematosus. Medicine. Feb 2018;46(2):84-92.

23. El Ghazali R, Bouziane H, Moudatir M, Echchilali K, Alaoui F, El Kabli HAnaemia during systemic lupus erythematosus: about 96 cases in a series of 184 cases. La Revue de Médecine Interne. june 2014;35:A89.

24. Echchilali K, Rihani N, Aboudib F, Moudatir M, Alaoui FZ, Elkabli H. Systemic lupus erythematosus and infection - 117 cases. La Revue de Médecine Interne. June 2013;34:A53.

25. Rees F, Doherty M, Grainge M, Davenport G, Lanyon P, Zhang W. The incidence and prevalence of systemic lupus erythematosus in the UK, 1999-2012. Annals of the Rheumatic Diseases. Jan 2016;75(1):136-41

APPENDIXES

Appendix 1: Classification criteria for systemic lupus erythematosus of the American College of Rheumatology {ACR) modified in 1997

1982 criteria modified in 1997 for the classification of systemic lupus erythematosus
Malaria rash Discoid lupus Photosensitivity Oral ulcers Non-erosive arthritis of at least two peripheral joints Pleurisy or pericarditis Kidney damage (proteinuria > 0.5 g d-1 or >+++or cellular cylinders) Convulsions or psychosis Hematological disorders : haemolytic anaemia or leukopenia (< 4,000 mm-3 on at least 2 occasions) or lymphopenia (< 1,500 mm-3 on at least 2 occasions) or thrombocytopenia (< 100,000 mm-3) in the absence of drug-related causes Immunological abnormality : anti-native DNA antibodies or anti-Smou antibodies high serum level of anticardiolipin IgG or M or positive standardised test for a circulating anticoagulant or false syphilitic serology (for at least 6 months) Antinuclear antibodies by immunofluorescence (in the absence of inducing drug)

Appendix 2: SLEDAI-SELENA

Score	Manifestations	Definitions
8	Convulsion	Recent onset. Exclusion of metabolic, infectious or other causes. medicinal products
8	Psychosis	Disturbance of normal activity associated with a severe alteration in the perception of reality, including hallucinations, incoherence, impoverished thought content, illogical reasoning, bizarre, disorganised or catatonic behaviour. Includes: hallucinations, incoherence, impoverished thought content, illogical reasoning, bizarre, disorganised or catatonic behaviour, or drug-induced.
8	Damage brain.	Impairment of mental functions with problems of orientation, memory or other, of sudden onset fluctuating course. Includes: disturbances of consciousness with reduced ability to concentrate, inability to pay attention, plus at least 2 of the following: perceptual disturbances, incoherent speech, insomnia or daytime sleepiness, increase in the number of hours of sleep per day. or reduced psychomotor activity.
8	Visual disorders	Retinal involvement in lupus. Includes: dysoric nodules, retinal haemorrhages, serous exudates or choroidal haemorrhages, optic neuritis. Exclusion of hypertensive, infectious or drug-induced causes.
8	Cranial nerves	New-onset sensory or motor neuropathy affecting a cranial nerve
8	Headache.	Severe, persistent headache, which may be migrainous but resistant to major analgesics.
8	STROKE	Recent cerebrovascular accident. Arteriosclerosis excluded.
8	Vasculitis.	Ulcerations, gangrene, painful digital nodules, peri-nail infarcts or histological or arteriographic evidence of vasculitis.
4	Arthritis	More than 2 painful joints with local inflammatory signs (pain, swelling or joint effusion).
4	Myositis.	Proximal muscle pain/weakness associated with CPK and/or aldolase, or electromyographic changes or biopsy showing signs of vasculitis.
4	Urinary cylinders	Red blood cell cylinders.
4	Haematuria.	> 5 g/field in the absence lithiasis, infection or other cause.
4	Proteinuria	> 0.5 GR/24 hours. Recent onset or recent increase of more than 0.5 g/24 hours.
4	Pyuria	> 5 GB/field in absence infection.
2	New rash	Recent appearance or recurrence of an inflammatory skin rash.
2	Alopecia.	Recent appearance or recurrence of patchy or diffuse alopecia.
2	Ulcers mucous	Recent appearance or recurrence oral or nasal ulcers.
2	Pleurisy	Chest pain of pleural origin with rubbing or effusion or pleural thickening.
2	Pericarditis.	Pericardial pain with at least one of the following symptoms: rubbing, effusion or electrographic or ultrasound confirmation.
2	[illegible] additional information	Decrease in CH50, C3 or C4< the lower laboratory normal.
2	Rise in anti DNA	Positive> 25% by the Farr test or level > laboratory normal.
1	Fever	> 38°C in the absence of an infectious cause.
1	Thrombocytopenia	< 100,000 platelets/mm3.
1	Leukopenia	< 3,000 WBC/mm3 in the absence of drug-induced causes.

SUMMARY

Systemic lupus erythematosus (SLE) is a non-organ-specific autoimmune disease. Male lupus is rarer but is considered to be more serious and more prone to complications. Our series identified the most common forms of disease developed during the course of male SLE: rheumatological manifestations (mainly arthralgia) were present in all patients, followed by mucocutaneous manifestations mainly malar rash and photosensitivity), which were present in 81% of patients. Renal involvement was present in 71.4% of patients. We found a high prevalence of cardiac and pleural manifestations in men. Fifteen male patients (71.4%) had a SLEDAI score of 11 or above, indicating high to very high disease activity. Infectious complications were dominated by pneumonitis and urinary tract infections. Non-infectious complications were mainly adverse effects of treatment, particularly corticosteroids.

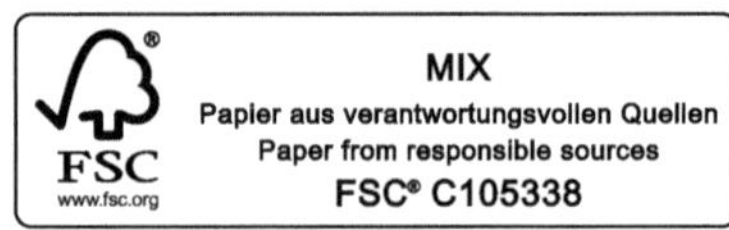

Printed by Books on Demand GmbH, Norderstedt / Germany